CH01455143

The 100

Powerful Affirmations

for Life Coaching

Condition Your Mind to Give the Most Powerful Advice To Each of Your Clients...

Jason Thomas

Copyright © 2016 WorldAffirmations.com All Rights Reserved.

No part of this publication may be reproduced, distributed, or transmitted in any form or by any means, including photocopying, recording, or other electronic or mechanical methods, or by any information storage and retrieval system without the prior written permission of the publisher, except in the case of very brief quotations embodied in critical reviews and certain other noncommercial uses permitted by copyright law.

WorldAffirmations.com

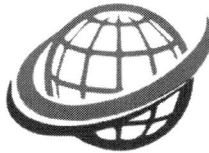

Do You Know **Exactly** How Affirmations Change Lives?

We'd like to give you a **FREE** copy of our book: *Affirmations Will Change Your Life*, available only & exclusively at WorldAffirmations.com.

Affirmations Will Change Your Life gives you step-by-step actions on why you need to use the power of affirmations in your daily life. It's also the precursor to all of WorldAffirmations.com's *Most Powerful Affirmations Series*.

This title is not available on Amazon, iBooks or Nook. It's only available at WorldAffirmations.com.

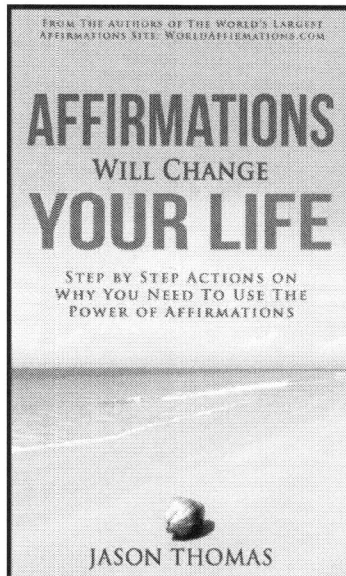

FROM THE AUTHORS OF THE WORLD'S LARGEST
AFFIRMATIONS SITE: WORLDAFFIRMATIONS.COM

AFFIRMATIONS
WILL CHANGE
YOUR LIFE
STEP BY STEP ACTIONS ON
WHY YOU NEED TO USE THE
POWER OF AFFIRMATIONS

JASON THOMAS

Table of Contents

Introduction

You are now taking the first steps to achieving fulfillment and happiness by becoming the architect of your own reality.

Imagine that with a few moments each day, you could begin the powerful transformation toward complete control of your life simply through affirmations.

You can begin that powerful transformation right now!

You will be able to release all fear and doubt simply because you know that you can. You can utilize this simple, proven technique to regain the lost comforts of joy, love, fulfillment and absolutely any other area of your life you want to improve.

You have the ability to unlock your full inner-potential and achieve your ultimate goals. This is the age-old secret of the financial elite, world-class scholars, and Olympic champions. For example, when you watch the Olympics you'll find one common consistency in all of the champions. Many, if not most, will close their eyes for a moment then clearly visualize & affirm to themselves completing the event flawlessly just before starting. Then they win gold medals, and become champions. These crisp affirmations are used by the most accomplished and fulfilled people in history. That's merely one example of how the real power of affirmation can elevate you above any of life's challenges.

You must believe and repeat affirmations each day, adding a few as you memorize them. If the thoughts and ideas that we affirm are not true in reality, a dynamic tension is created between your perceived reality and your psyche. This presence of dynamic tension causes imbalance between your psyche and perceived reality. Your consciousness will work to get back in tune with the universe to resolve the tension. There are two simple ways to ease this tension. You must work with the universe in order to make your affirmations become true. As you choose to continue affirming, your mind and body will seek to balance this inequality with the universe by transforming your environment to match your declarations of truth. Sooner than later, you will find yourself taking positive and decisive action that you never imagined possible, as your perceptions naturally align with your true reality.

As you begin to attune yourself to the positive energy around you it will become easier and easier to create the world you perceive.

Affirmation isn't intended to make you delude yourself or simply throw a blanket over the negative aspects of your life. The intention is to magnify your focus on the positive reality you desire and the possibility thereof. Affirmation will not force you to get up from your chair and magically start a multi-billion dollar business in a single day. But, affirmation will help you take control of your motivation and release doubt, giving you the power to pave the steps in front of you, as you stride confidently toward your manifesting goals.

You are now striding confidently toward manifesting your goals!

Many affirmations in this book may stick with you or touch you in a special way. Please feel free to take them into your daily life and use them. There is no reason to stick rigidly to the use of any particular set, or to limit your use of them. Find out what works for you. Chances are if it makes you feel positive and empowered, it's working wonders.

These affirmations are for use everywhere. As you begin to use them, you will find yourself remembering certain ones in certain stressful situations. This is your consciousness learning to replace negative patterns with positive affirmation. When you feel this begin to happen, don't worry! The tingling means it's working.

By utilizing these affirmations, you are training your consciousness to work in tandem with the Universe's natural flow of energy. This is how we are naturally designed to function as happy, healthy beings. Unfortunately, the complexity of the world has made it more difficult to find the natural creative harmony we each have inside of us. Negative thinking goes against the larger natural order of the universe, and will unravel along with those who harbor it.

An affirmation is defined as, "A positive, confident, and forceful statement of fact or belief." Anything you think or say is a statement of fact or belief. It's the forceful confidence that gives affirmation its power.

If you want to see positive change now, you'll find the quickest path to fulfillment with affirmation. There is no time to spend on loss, negativity, and defeat when you can be achieving tangible, historically proven results with minimum time and effort invested.

Consider the following your prescription for results.

1. Review the following list of affirmations in full.

2. Pick Five to Ten affirmations that powerfully resonate with you.

3. Repeat several times a day at different intervals. (Minimum Five times a day)

4. Use anything available to remind you during a busy day: a daily planner, phone alarm, etc.

5. Do this consistently for Ninety Days.

At the end of these ninety days, you will notice, without doubt, that less and less is happening to you in your life by default. Then you can repeat with the next subject that you wish to make powerful change in your life with.

Enjoy!

The 100 Most Powerful

Affirmations for Life Coaching

I pass on what I know to others and enrich their lives...

I look forward to every day of my life...

I am able to share the power and strength I have as a personality...

I have learned active listening and know its value...

I am the perfect life coach for those who seek advice...

I am powerful because I listen as well as talk...

I am able to make other people's lives fulfilled and happy...

I know the direction of my life and can steer others to finding their own direction...

I am loyal and people trust my judgment...

I have much to give others and enjoy sharing my knowledge...

I know the secrets of success and get joy from sharing them...

I choose to be a coach because it helps people get their lives on track...

I am good at sharing great news and enjoy the challenge...

The power that I have makes getting up each day worthwhile...

I have everything that I ever wanted in life...

I am able to show people how to achieve their dreams...

I have the ability to change lives...

I am a strong teacher and mentor...

I give my secrets to those who recognize my abilities...

I am able to share all of my ideas with others...

I am strong in character and help others to find their own strengths...

I am able to make money from being myself...

I have the exact life I want to have...

I have the power to change lives for the better...

I have all the resources I need to help others...

I am grateful for the strength of character I was born with...

I am a source of great inspiration for others...

I am always looking for new ways to make the lives of others better...

I am a great source of energy for others...

I know how to bring out the best in people...

I am gifted with being able to help others...

I am rich because I am good at what I do...

I make my living being able to improve other people's lives...

I am confident and able to help anyone who chooses to be helped...

I can turn negative people into positive successes...

I know how to switch on all the right switches...

I am able to make people think about their approaches to life...

I am stronger than others...

I have a wealth of inner strength...

I am always filled with enthusiasm...

I know that I love the work that I do...

I am able to use something I love to help others...

I can make people fulfill their dreams...

I understand how people need to change in order to win...

I have no doubts in myself because I know my way is right...

I can teach people to use their own inner resources to get rich...

I am self-motivated and need no one to push me...

I am able to give people good value for money...

I know that my advice is sound and helps others...

I have confidence in my own abilities...

I am able to put forward ideas that others don't think of...

I know how to be successful and enjoy the benefits of success...

I train people to train themselves...

I have no problem teaching others because I know my own disciplines...

I am disciplined and motivated in my work...

I have resources at my disposal at all times...

I am positive in my approach...

I am without a doubt the best at what I do...

I can give people exactly what they want...

I am an active listener and use this to help others...

I can turn people's lives around for the better...

I give my clients value for money...

I am able to take on difficult cases and make them simple...

I have no doubt in my ability to change lives...

I am doing the job that my heart is happy with...

I am the best coach out there...

I am completely honest in my dealings with people...

I know that people trust me to empower their lives...

I have great results from the work that I do...

I have a powerful mind that enriches my life...

I can enrich the lives of others...

I am able to give others as much as I have given myself...

I look in the mirror and see a successful smile...

I live the exact life my dreams were made of...

I know where I am going in life and help others to find direction...

I am able to walk into a room and change people's attitudes...

I convince others that they have the power to change their lives...

I am able to pass on to others the great powers I was born with...

I know I can trust my intuition...

I know that my common sense tells me what I need to do...

I have an inner voice that guides me toward success...

I have no doubts in my motives and this keeps me on track...

I can give people their dreams and make them happen...

I live my dream because I know how to...

I am never short of ideas to help those seeking out their dreams...

I make people powerful and happy...

I turn people into superstars...

I am able to watch my clients start to understand success...

I am a powerhouse of positivity...

I love what I do and others see this and want the same things...

I know that anyone is capable of catching their dreams...

I am able to be a mentor to people looking for a better life...

I am grateful for the powers given to me to help others succeed...

I am always ready to change someone's life for the better...

I take the lead and let clients learn how to do the same...

I love my job as it gives me everything I ever wanted...

I train people to train themselves...

I am a great coach because I believe in what I have to give...

I know my clients lives are improved by what I do...

I am a coach because I know the difference I can make to other people's lives...

The 100 Most Powerful

Affirmations for Mindfulness

I have learned through mindfulness to use all of my senses...

I am able to communicate with others on an equal basis because I am mindful of the differences between us...

I will always be mindful of the food that I eat...

I am enriched by my mindful attitude toward others...

I am mindful of my moments in life and enjoy them to the maximum...

I am able to enjoy everything about life because I miss nothing...

I know my moments are filled with new experiences...

I have learned that looking back gives no value to my life...

I am planted in the moment and that enriches my life...

I know that mindful people are happier people...

I am aware that mindfulness is the answer to end problems...

I am mindful of the importance of humility...

I appreciate everything that life offers me...

I can enjoy all of the wonders of nature as I observe them...

I am richer in my life than ever before...

I know that nature offers me much happiness...

I love the sunlight that penetrates into the recesses of my mind...

I am able to look at the raindrops and see rainbows of opportunity...

I am lucky to wake each day and to be conscious of everything around me...

I love life because I live each moment of it in awareness...

I have more than my fair share of happiness because my mind is peaceful...

I have closed the door to past regrets...

I do not care about the future, but assure it by living in the moment...

I am able to appreciate the smile of a child and embrace it...

I can hold my head up high, knowing that my stature is measured only by my understanding...

I love to watch the changing of the seasons and embrace the colors...

I know that my senses are alive when I smell the rain...

I am happy to watch the flowers push through the Earth in spring...

I am mindful of everything around me...

I know that mindfulness has ended all of my doubts in life...

I am aware of my own beauty and do not measure it against other people's interpretation of who I should be...

I am aware of others and have learned the gift of listening...

I close my eyes and I still feel the ambiance because my other senses are alive...

I am able to hold my hand against a leaf and feel the connection of touch...

I am divinely happy through my own mindful ways...

I live a life of abundance and enjoy it to the full...

I am a child of nature and embrace nature as part of me...

I am at peace with the child inside me...

I can recognize the difference between failure and success...

I can see and hear things that other people don't notice...

I have the ability to feel emotions and to use them to learn...

I am not closed off to the potential life offers me...

I keep myself aware and awareness enhances my life...

I am aware that my happiness is a product of my mindfulness...

I keep myself happy by enjoying awareness...

I am a valuable human being who gains energy from mindfulness...

I meditate and discover inner riches I never thought possible...

I am wonderfully mindful because I was well taught...

I use mindfulness in all of my relationships...

I am able to be mindful instead of argumentative and the results are positive...

I make friends easily because my attitude to life is flexible...

I never hold grudges because yesterday's pain is gone...

I am able to smile in the face of problems, knowing mindfulness will give me the answers...

I am mindful that I can become anyone I wish to become...

I have developed a friendship and bond between mind and body...

I know that I can still my mind when stillness provides me with the energy I need...

I am able to go through life with a positive attitude...

I hold each moment in my life dearly...

I have this moment to be the best person I can be...

I have learned to stem the flow of my thoughts to the present...

I am grounded and happy in this moment...

I taste the fruits from the trees and enjoy their refreshment...

I smell the air and am delighted by it...

I touch a leaf and feel its fragility...

I see the skies and am closer to spiritual awareness...

I am able to use my mind in each second to make that second count...

I live my life to the full through mindfulness...

I never worry about tomorrow...

I never concern myself with past events...

I meditate in the moment...

I have found great peace through knowing life's moments pass too quickly for regret...

I am mindful of all the good things in life...

I know mindfulness makes me a more complete person...

I sing the song of completeness and enjoy each note...

I am able to taste the sea through the power of thought...

I am alive and grateful for each moment...

I give my best to each passing moment of time...

I never watch my clock as time passes without my intervention...

I know and respect myself...

I am mindful of the gifts life has given me...

I love my life through mindfulness...

I am careful with my words and deeds...

I take my time to enjoy each moment of my life...

I am who I am and this moment in my life is the best ever...

I can feel the warmth of love caress my body...

I love who I am and who I have become...

I am mindful of my breathing in the energy of life...

I always stop to smell the roses...

I know there is not a moment in my life that is wasted...

I give everything I am to this moment in time...

I am capable of stemming thoughts that detract from this moment...

I am positive in my outlook toward life...

I have everything a human being could ever want, need or desire...

I am happy and contented in this very moment...

I look into the mirror and see a happy person looking back...

I am thankful for the people who make my life enjoyable...

I am grateful for the chance to be who I am...

I make my moments count as productive and happy...

I am aware of people around me and have learned empathy...

I am a better person than I was yesterday...

The 100 Most Powerful

Affirmations for Motivation

I will go out and be successful today...

I am constantly accomplishing new goals all the time...

I have endless energy and motivation...

I enjoy new challenges and face them head-on...

I am always moving toward my dreams...

I am important and my work makes a difference...

I am a wildly motivated person...

I always get things done on time...

I make the most efficient use of my time...

I am a very ambitious and driven person...

I am viewed by others as a highly motivated person...

I stay motivated for the entirety of any project...

I will find my motivation when I need it...

I have a bottomless pool of motivational energy...

I become more and more passionate about my goals all the time...

I am always ready to get started...

I am a naturally motivated person...

I make passionate motivation a part of my daily life...

I am motivated more by each action that I take...

I work hard each day to realize my dreams...

I constantly bring my goals closer to my grasp...

I know how to keep myself motivated and interested...

I am more motivated to succeed than ever before...

I am self-motivated in everything I do...

I easily stay focused and on track...

I have the opportunity to be more successful today...

I am making today as productive as possible...

I will accomplish everything I set out to do today...

I love to set new goals for myself...

I find it easy to work toward my goals and dreams...

I have a motivation that expands with my workload...

I am unable to run out of motivation...

I will let my energy help others to stay motivated...

I like to encourage others to work hard by setting the example...

I have no fear of taking on new challenges...

I will embrace my day and use my time to the fullest...

I am pleased to find new goals to challenge myself with...

I have a direct path to my dreams through hard work...

I will make my dreams a reality no matter what it takes...

I am constantly making strides toward greatness...

I know that my work in the world makes it a better place...

I have a significant and necessary impact on the world around me...

I will allow my motivation to help enrich the lives of others...

I easily meet and beat expectations for my work...

I am motivated, punctual, and hard-working...

I will not let failure be an option...

I do not know how to give up...

I will find ways to make myself more efficient...

I have the power to increase my capacity for work...

I am always finding new ways to better manage my time...

I will stay driven because it is naturally how I am...

I have no limit to my ambition...

I enjoy having lots of things to do...

I set an example of motivation and action for others to follow...

I like to do the tough jobs first...

I am at maximum interest from the beginning to the end of a project...

I am a person who always steps forward to take action...

I get things done just because I see that they need to be done...

I never have trouble finding my motivation...

I am immensely satisfied by working toward my goals...

I am easily self-empowered by my affirmations...

I seize and work for every opportunity I see...

I make the most of every day that I get...

I will work until I am living my dreams...

I love to start working early so things get done sooner...

I am not slowed down by minor setbacks...

I am brimming with can-do energy...

I am motivated by an endless energy that the universe gives to me...

I speak words that motivate and empower others...

I find new reasons to work for my goals each day...

I am passionate about the accomplishments I am creating...

I am constantly ready to begin new projects...

I always have room on my plate for more things to do...

I enjoy working on multiple projects at once...

I like to do things myself because I know they get done right...

I have a constant desire to be accomplishing something...

I am always reaching out to get closer to my goals...

I enjoy goals that are challenging to reach...

I have a habit of increasing my work efficiency...

I enjoy helping others get things done...

I am naturally moving all the time...

I work hard, fast, and efficiently...

I am not deterred by difficult to reach goals...

I am known for my hard work and dedication...

I make hard work fun and rewarding...

I feel deep satisfaction when I am working on a project...

I have enough motivation that I can share with others...

I have a powerful drive to succeed...

I am always focused on completing things perfectly...

I see opportunities everywhere and I take them...

I have the power to make my dreams a reality through hard work...

I raise the bar for my accomplishments daily...

I look back on each day with a sense of accomplishment...

I am never wasting time...

I feel a deep fulfillment when I work toward my goals...

I will work until my life is everything I desire...

I am able to mold the world around me with little effort...

I find most tasks easy and simple to complete...

I am the one who people call on when they need something done right...

I often enjoy work more than rest...

Thank You!

I want to sincerely thank you for reading this book!

Let me finish though by saying the work isn't done here. These must be put to use repetitively, and on a daily basis to see changes in your life.

Remember to follow the ninety-day plan outlined in the introduction to maximize your results.

Can I ask you for a very quick favor? Can you leave a review on our Amazon.com detail page to tell us about your progress and how you enjoyed the book?

We take the time to go over each review personally, and your feedback in invaluable to us as writers, and others that wish to see the same change in their lives as you:)

Thank You!

28240003R00051

Printed in Poland
by Amazon Fulfillment
Poland Sp. z o.o., Wrocław